7 Day Tea Cleanse Diet Plan

How to Choose Your Detox Teas, Boost Your Metabolism, Lose 10 Pounds a Week, Flush out Toxins and Improve Your Health

Clayton West

Table of Contents

Introduction

We've all heard of the detox plans that claim to cleanse you with just a drink and most of us are well aware that a liquid-only diet is not going to sustain our bodies for very long. But the tea cleanse diet, or teatox as it is known, is more than just swilling a few drinks every day. The tea cleanse diet is a far gentler method simply because instead of replacing meals with drinks, herbal teas are added to a clean food diet. This means that unlike many other detox diets, the tea cleanse allows you to eat real food as well.

The potent powers of tea are known and experienced worldwide. Studies carried out across the entire world have shown that tea has the ability to lower the risk of heart disease and stroke, lower your blood pressure and to stimulate you mentally. In addition, tea can also help you to keep your weight down and your energy levels up.

When it comes to detoxifying the body, tea alone is not enough. There's no one single food, drink or herb that can cure the body of any diseases or ailments, or to detoxify the body. Instead, tea must be drunk in addition to a healthy clean diet. Black and green teas are full of vital antioxidants and these help to boost the detoxification process.

Antioxidants work by reducing free radicals and oxidative stress in the body, the combination that causes inflammation and can even cause a mutation to your DNA strain that can lead to many chronic diseases, including cancer.
Of course, as well as the pure green and black teas, you will come across many other varieties, including those that are branded as detox teas. These include extra ingredients that aid detoxification, including herbs that support the liver, like:

- Ginger
- Lemongrass
- Milk thistle
- Dandelion

The liver is the main organ in charge of the detoxifying process and when it becomes blocked and sluggish, it cannot do its job and that means waste is not being eliminated from your body properly. Ginger is one of the best at reducing the oxidative stress on the liver, helping to work more efficiently and effectively at keeping the toxins out of your body.

This book will tell you how to use the tea cleanse diet to jumpstart your metabolism and lose up to 10 lbs. in just one week. Will also give you a few recipes to try, recipes that will give you the idea of what foods to eat while you are on the 7-day tea cleanse and afterward. Because you will be eating real food and healthy smoothies as well, you won't get the hunger pangs that so often accompany detox diets and you will be getting all of the nutrients and vitamins that your body needs.

Ready to try? Here's how to drink tea and drop pounds.

Chapter 1: Why Tea Cleanse?

Why do any cleanse? Every day our bodies are subjected to an onslaught of toxins that can build up and begin to make us feel lethargic. We suffer from constant headaches, other aches and pains and a feeling of malaise that we often can't put our fingers on. Sadly, many people don't even know where to begin with a detox let alone actually doing one and those of us that do look into them are often scared silly by what they entail.

One of the best and easiest ways to cleanse your body is through tea and here's how:

Green Tea

Most people have heard of how wonderful green tea is, of the powers of healing it contains. Green tea is packed with antioxidants and vital vitamins and some of its best features include:

- Fat burning – the antioxidants help to speed up your metabolism and this means you burn fat as energy even when you aren't active

- Improves immune response – this helps you to better fight off flu, colds, and other troublesome illness

- Fights disease – many studies show that green tea can help to prevent and fight cancer, diabetes, and arthritis

- Hydrating – green tea is as hydrating, if not more so, than plain old water

- Neurological help – green tea has been shown to help prevent or slow down neurological and degenerative diseases like Alzheimer's

Japanese Matcha Tea

If you thought green tea was good, welcome to Matcha. Just one cup of this is the equivalent of 10 cups of green tea. Key benefits are:

- Cancer preventative – because of the high levels of catechin, antioxidants which actively seek and destroy dangerous free radicals

- Heart disease preventative – because it lowers levels of LDL cholesterol, the bad type

- Fat burner – because it increases a process called thermogenesis from 8-10% to 35-43%

- Neurological benefits – because it contains L-theanine. This is an amino acid that provides more help with neurological activities.

Refresh Tea

When you use tea to detox with, it will always be in two parts. First, you start the day with a refresh tea and then you end the day with the colon cleanse tea. The morning tea is designed to help replace the electrolytes and vitamins that are lost through the evening tea and, if you don't drink it, you will not realize the true potential of the tea cleanse. The refresh tea should contain ingredients that are high in vitamins and antioxidants as an absolute basic and you can add other ingredients to the tea, like:

- Ginseng
- Acai berry
- Spirulina
- Barley grass

If you find that the flavor is not quite what you expect and hard to stomach, you can also add any of these:

- ☐ Lemon juice
- ☐ Organic honey
- ☐ Stevia
- ☐ Ginger powder
- ☐ Mulberries

Colon Cleanse Tea

In order for the detox to work, you have to get rid of the buildup of toxins and heavy metals in your body. The colon cleanse tea should contain one key ingredient – Senna leaf. Senna is a natural laxative and the blend that you make up, if you make your own, is important to increase how effective it is. Add some of these to your Senna leaf tea:

- ☐ Dandelion plant
- ☐ Dried orange peel
- ☐ Lemongrass
- ☐ Nettle leaf
- ☐ Liquorice root

All of these flavor the tea nicely and increase the benefits. Of course, you can buy specially made t-bags but using loose tea or making your own blends is often recommended for better effect.

Chapter 2: How does Tea Cleanse Work?

No doubt you have read about or even tried other cleanses, only to find that they do not work. The tea cleanse is something very different because you eat food, real food, something that other cleanses forbid. Being able to eat food as well means that your metabolism remains high, an important thing if you are looking to drop the pounds. So, how does the tea cleanse work?

Aside from the fact that you will be taking in fewer calories overall, the fact that you are drinking proper teas, drinking tea-based smoothies and eating real food means that your body is getting a proper dose of goodness, all the vital minerals, and vitamins that you need for your body to work properly.

The benefits of the tea cleanse are numerous and much of this is down to the high levels of antioxidant found in the teas. These are called polymerized polyphenols and they help to stop the body from absorbing fat by up to 20%. Here are the ways in which the tea cleanse works to benefit your body:

- Lower blood pressure. If you drink around 120 ml of tea every day, you will lower your risk of high blood pressure by up to 46%.

- Stronger bones – the catechins in some teas have been shown to boost bone growth and slow the speed at which bone cells break down. A separate study has shown that theaflavin, one of the antioxidants in tea, slows the function of DNA methyltransferase, an enzyme that attacks bone tissue as we age.

- Stronger immune system – people who drink around 20 oz. of black tea every day produce up to 5 times more of one of the key parts of the infection protections system in their bodies.

- Slow down aging – Studies have shown that an extract of white tea may be able to help slow down the appearance of wrinkle and give your skin a younger look.

- Less stress, better sleep – no doubt you already know that chamomile tea is one of the best to help you sleep but other herbal teas can also help you to relax and sleep better. Rooibos tea has a number of compounds that lower stress, help you to sleep and, even better, lower the ability of the cells to store fat.

- Lower risk of cancer - EGCG is an active ingredient in green tea that can trigger off a cycle that can kill cancer cells in the mouth. It can also build up the capability to protect in the normal cells that are around those cancer cells.

On top of all these amazing health benefits, you also get the added benefit of a clean colon, and a real spring in the step when you ditch your usual drinks in favor of tea.

Chapter 3: The Principles of the Tea Cleanse

Believe it or not, tea can give you back full control over your health your body, your weight and, perhaps more importantly, your mind. In some countries, tea is as common as water, with vending machines selling, not cans of soda but cups of tea. When you make the switch over to tea, you will not believe the changes in yourself. Not only are you drinking something incredibly thirst-quenching and nourishing, you are changing your life and your body for the better.

You already know what tea can do for you in terms of health, now it's time to look at the principles of the tea cleanse so you know what to expect and how to go about the 7-day tea cleanse diet:

Meals

Every day, you will have two meals, including a tea cleanse smoothie and this will take anywhere between 800 and 1700 calories every single day off your intake, without affecting your energy levels in any adverse way or without leaving you hungry. Each meal will be packed with nutrition, will be easy and quick to make and made with real whole foods.

Hot Tea

Each day you will drink 5 cups of hot nourishing tea. Each of the teas will be selected to provide you with the maximum level of benefit at the time it is needed. You will drink:

- One cup of metabolism-burning tea, designed to boost your fat burners

☐ One cup of flat-belly tea, to cut the bloat and help to fight off inflammation

☐ Two cups of fat-block tea, once before you have your midday smoothie and once before your dinner. These help to reduce hunger, shrink down the fat cells and stop you from gaining weight

☐ One up of stress-busting tea to ensure that your focus is clear and you get a better night's sleep.

Smoothies

Each day, you will get to drink one cool and deliciously creamy tea-based smoothie. These are designed to help fill you up with nutrients that melt the fat away.

Start Your Day

Begin your day with a walk, everyday. Not a pound-the-pavement walk, but a gentle one walk to kick-start the ingredients in your morning cup of tea.

At 7 AM, you will have 1 or 2 cups of metabolism tea. Choose from:

☐ Green
☐ Yerba mate   Green
☐ Goji
☐ Kola nut
☐ Oolong

Follow this up with a walk lasting between 10 and 30 minutes - outdoors is best.

At 10 AM, drink one cup of fat-blocker tea – choose from:

- ☐ White
- ☐ Black
- ☐ Green
- ☐ Rooibos
- ☐ Barberry
- ☐ Pu-erh

White or Rooibos

At 12 noon, drink an 8 oz. smoothie – see recipe ideas later on

At 3 PM, you will drink a cup of the flat belly tea – choose from:

- ☐ Mint
- ☐ Ginger
- ☐ Hibiscus
- ☐ Bilberry
- ☐ Fennel
- ☐ Lemon

Fennel

At 6 PM chose another cup of fat-blocker tea from the list above

White

At 7 PM you will have your tea cleanse meal. A few recipe ideas are given at the end of this book

At 9 PM drink one up of stress-busting tea – choose from:

- ☐ Kava kava
- ☐ Ashwagandha
- ☐ Hops
- ☐ Rooibos
- ☐ Passionflower
- ☐ Lemon balm
- ☐ Chamomile and lavender
- ☐ Valerian

Lemon Balm

Later on, I will go into more detail as to how and why this combination works.

Chapter 4: What are Toxins?

The detox diet is not a new thing but the last few years have seen them become the in-thing to do. Everywhere you look there are pills, powders, juice detox, salt detox - anything you can possibly think of, all claiming to release the toxins from your body. That's all well and good and the tea cleanse diet does exactly the same thing. But, unlike all those other detox diets, I'm actually going to tell you what these toxins are and the damage they do to your body. If you don't understand toxins, then there is little point in you doing a detox because you won't understand what is harming you and what isn't.

So, What Are These Toxins?

When you look for a definition of toxin, you will find that it is quite vague. The definition in the Merriam-Webster dictionary states that:

"A toxin is a poisonous substance that is a specific product of the metabolic activities of a living organism and is usually very unstable, notably toxic when introduced into the tissues, and typically capable of inducing antibody formation."

In simple terms, a toxin is a substance or matter that can harm you. So why is the definition so vague? Because there are, literally thousands of different types of toxins and each one has its own effects, detrimental or otherwise. To clarify things, we break toxins down into 3 separate categories – internal, eternal and toxic behavior.

Internal Toxins

The human body is a wonderful thing. It can defend itself, repair itself and even poison itself! We already produce a certain level of toxins in our bodies just by living and breathing. But, we also have our own internal processes that get rid of these naturally occurring toxins and stop them from building up.

Our body burns energy on an almost constant basis so that dying cells can be replaced and tissue rebuilt. Because of this, we are also making a lot of waste in the form of internal toxins, all of which have to be broken down, recycled where needed and the rest eliminated. The problems occur when these toxins build up to a level that is harmful. The body is always producing these toxins and it doesn't get the time that it needs to deal with the buildup. Instead, the excess toxins, the ones they can't deal with are pushed to one side and they are left alone to cause havoc on the surrounding cells and organs. Without some much-needed help, they begin to clog up your system and this results in the body using up more energy just to function normally and this leaves you feeling worn out.

Some of the things that can affect the levels of internal toxins are basic things like medications. Antacids, for example, can slow your digestion down and result in a poor absorption rate of vitamins. If you use Tylenol long term your liver will stop detoxifying itself. In fact, use of Tylenol on a long-term basis can cause liver failure.

Signs that internal toxins are building up

- Chronic infection, like dysbiosis of the GI tract and sinusitis

- Allergic reactions – delayed and immediate onset. The common ones include corn eggs, dairy and gluten allergies

- High liver enzymes

External Toxins

So, with our bodies working like well-oiled machinery, why do we get such high levels of toxins? Put simply, although the body can mostly cope with the toxins we produce ourselves, we have to add external toxins into the mix as well. These are toxins that can be absorbed or ingested into the body. So many people believe that all of our toxins come from food but they couldn't be more wrong. A certain amount do but there are other places, like the deodorant or shampoo that you use, right down to the water you drink. Some examples are:

- Environmental, such as smog, debris, smoke, etc.

- Mercury – in some fish that you eat

- Lead – some canned goods, blinds, old paint

- Aluminum – in deodorants, antacids, and antiperspirant

- Mold – inhaled when damp rooms are not properly ventilated, like bathrooms or basements

- Poor air – inhaled from rooms that are not ventilated or are badly maintained ventilation

- Food and water that has been contaminated

- Chemicals – house cleaning products and pet products

- Phthalates and bisphenol A – in soft plastics

- UV radiation

Toxic Behaviors

Most people associate toxin with physical products or elements but things that you do can also have a negative effect on toxin levels. For example, if you are constantly in contact with chemicals, you can expect higher levels of toxins but nobody associates working long hours with the same thing. Stress and overwork will eventually take its toll on you - excessive stress tends to lead to bad eating habits, anxiety, lethargy and depression and all of this can lead to a number of chronic illnesses.

Other toxic behaviors

- Overeating
- A bad diet
- Smoking
- Excessive use of drugs, prescribed, over the counter or otherwise
- Excessive use of alcohol
- Lethargy
- Lack of self-control

Chapter 5: Detoxification for Rejuvenation

It's no secret that green tea is considered to be one of the healthiest drinks on earth. The trouble is, most people hate the taste – until they get used to it. Like many things, it takes a little perseverance and, eventually, you won't be able to do without it. Green tea is one of the best teas to include in any detox regime, especially one for rejuvenation.

Green tea is made in a specific way using just the two top buds and leaves of the Camellia Sinensis plant. On occasion, other ingredients are added to these in the drying process. The leaves are dried to stop them from fermenting and this stops enzyme activity. The next step is to steam the leaves for about 90 seconds before moving on to the final processing stage.

Before you get stuck into a vat full of green tea, you should be aware of a few things:

- It has caffeine in it so drinking too much will affect the way you sleep

- It is a stimulant and that means your kidneys get stimulated too. Expect to be on and out of the bathroom!

- It contains tannins which block correct absorption of folic acid and iron so, if you are pregnant or planning to get pregnant, you should not drink it in high amounts

As well as green tea, there are a number of foods that you should be eating as way of detoxing to rejuvenate your body. How do you know if you need rejuvenation? Ask yourself if you suffer from one or more of these:

- Fatigue
- Headaches
- Insomnia
- Depression
- Allergies
- Any one of a number of degenerative diseases that are due to exposure to toxins

If you do, then it's time to give your body what it needs. The following are seven vital foods that you should include in your diet to help your body detox and rejuvenate:

- Blueberries – these help to block the toxins from getting past the blood-brain barrier and entering the fatty tissues in your brain

- Cruciferous vegetables – like cabbage, broccoli, kale, spinach, cauliflower, etc. These have been proven to help neutralize damaging compounds that come from cigarette smoke. They also contain a specific compound that assists the liver in the production of enzymes that help with detoxification

- Carrots – these contain beta-carotene which is useful for cleansing heavy metals from your body

- Grapefruit - contains pectin which will bind to the heavy metals in your body and helps to neutralize them and safely eliminate them

- Lemons – contain vitamin C, which helps in the production of glutathione. This is what is used to help phase 2 detoxification of the liver keep up with phase 1 detoxification, thus cutting down on the risk of any negative effects from environmental toxins

- ☐ Onions – have been shown to cleanse your blood and help the respiratory tract to detoxify

- ☐ Seaweed – will bind to any radioactive waste and any heavy metals in your body and ensure that they are safely eliminated

A few more tips to help you detoxify for rejuvenation safely and effectively:

- ☐ Always buy organic food where you can.

- ☐ If you have to take nutritional supplements, ensure that they are high-quality ones.

- ☐ Make sure you exercise to help sweat the toxins out.

Chapter 6: 7 Day Tea Cleanse Diet Schedule Plan

When you do the 7-day tea cleanse diet, you will more than likely see some excellent results within the first 3 days. Many who have tried it have said that they lost, in just 7 days up to 3 inches off their waistlines. The tea cleanse is designed, not just around tea, but also around eating perfect food. This is an intense cleanse so please do not do this for any more than 7 days. However, during those 7 days, you are going to learn things about your body and you will learn how to get your body to strip the fat without even trying. You can also repeat this plan when you have a big event, like a wedding or a Christmas ball to attend. Here's how to do it and how it all works:

Teas

Chose one cup of tea, five times per day, from the above list. You will have two weight loss teas, one flat belly tea, and one stress buster tea.

Why this works

We all know about balanced diets – a proper one gives us the correct balance of nutrient for every day. Tea is the same in that you will be getting a balance of all the special properties contained in the different teas.

Meals

You will have a tea-based smoothie and a wonderfully tasty dinner but absolutely NO dessert.

Why this works:

On average, a man consumes approximately 2700 calories per day while a woman will consume between 1850 and 2200. On the tea cleanse, that will drop to around 1000 calories and that deficit means that a woman can drop around 4 lbs. in 10 days, just through calories, and a man will lose about 5. Obviously, we also have to factor in other things, like metabolic impact, how the tea makes fat cells shrink and how powerful the tea is at deflating you. You could lose as much as 14 lbs. in 7 days!

Smoothies

Every day you will have one delicious tea-based smoothie at lunchtime. As well as tasting gorgeous, these smoothies are designed to strip away fat as opposed to packing you full of sugar like some smoothies do.

Why this works

These smoothies are balanced to make sure your body gets all the nutrition it needs but without the calorie count. Green tea is normally the base and we know now that this is one of the healthiest drinks on the planet.

Cleanse Foods

For the 7 days that you are on the cleanse, you are going to have to make your own meals, which mean no eating out! Each of the meals that you will eat over the next week is going to be less than 500 calories and will consist of healthy fats, vegetables, protein and a small amount of fruit and grains. This might sound harsh but it is only for 7 days.

Why this Works

When you sleep, your metabolism decreases by around 35% and that means if you have unused carbohydrates in your system when you go to bed, they are highly likely to be turned into glucose. This will then get stored as fat in your body, the last thing you need. Fruit and grain product are the two main carbohydrate source.

Alcohol

No more than one alcoholic drink, every two days – wine is best

Why this Works:

Alcohol is full of calories so one of the quickest ways to cut empty calories out of your diet is to cut down or cut it out completely. Alcohol is also a toxin. When you drink a glass of wine or beer, your body kicks into burn-off mode to get rid of the calories as fast as it can and, to do that it will ignore all the other calories that came in with the alcohol. So if you drink while you are eating, the calories in the alcohol will be metabolized while the calories in the food get pushed into your fat cells.

Your Morning Ritual

A 10-30 minute walk every morning

Why this works:

Fasted exercise, i.e. exercise before your first food of the day, is far better at burning off fat than exercising later on. The key here is to exercise lightly before eating but do have a metabolism tea first as this will make the effects of the exercise much better. The reason behind this is that when you eat something, you provide your body with glycogen and this is what gets you through the day. When you exercise that glycogen has to be burnt off before it reaches your fat cells. But, if you exercise before you eat, your energy burning will come mostly from fat and that results in faster weight loss, up to 20% more in many cases.

Dessert

You can't have any for the next 7 days

Why this works:
By not eating after 7 PM at night your body is perfectly set for burning off the fat with your morning walk. And, that first cup of metabolism tea will provide you with double the effect over just a fast. Plus, most desserts are loaded with sugar, carbohydrate, and calories, not to mention bad fat.

If you are ready to change your life and change your body for the better, in the net chapter I will give you some ideas for smoothies and meals.

Chapter 7: Tea Cleanse Recipes

Smoothies

For all of these recipes, simply chuck the ingredients into your blender and give it a whiz until smooth and creamy.

Green Banana

- 1 ripe banana
- ½ cup milk
- ½ cup green tea
- 1 tbsp. agave syrup
- 1 tbsp. organic peanut butter
- 1 cup ice

Blueberry Monster

- ☐ 1 cup blueberries
- ☐ ½ cup Greek yogurt
- ☐ ½ cup green tea
- ☐ 1 tbsp. flaxseed
- ☐ 4 ice cubes

Big Orange Crush

- ¾ cup mango, frozen
- ½ cup green tea
- ½ cup carrot juice
- ½ cup Greek yogurt
- ½ cup water
- 1 tbsp. protein powder

Strawberry Papaya

- ☐ ¾ cup strawberries, frozen
- ☐ ¾ cup papaya, frozen
- ☐ ½ cup green tea
- ☐ ½ cup milk
- ☐ 1 tbsp. fresh mint leaves

Punchy Pineapple

- ☐ 1 cup pineapple, frozen
- ☐ ½ cup Greek yogurt
- ☐ ½ cup green tea
- ☐ ½ cup milk

Big Green Goddess

- ☐ ¼ pitted and peeled avocado
- ☐ 1 tbsp. organic honey
- ☐ 1 ripe banana
- ☐ ½ cup green tea
- ☐ ½ cup ice
- ☐ 1 scoop of protein powder

Optional ingredient – 1 tsp. ginger, fresh grated

Meals

Black Bean Omelet

Ingredients

- [ ] 14-16 oz. can drained black beans
- [ ] ¼ tsp. cumin
- [ ] Juice from one lime
- [ ] 8 eggs
- [ ] ½ cup + extra feta cheese
- [ ] Salt and pepper to taste
- [ ] Hot sauce to taste
- [ ] Bottled salsa

Method:

1. Put the beans, cumin, lime and a bit of hot sauce into your blender and whiz until you have something the consistency of refried beans – add water if necessary
2. Heat a little olive oil or butter in a pan
3. Beat two eggs with salt and pepper and add them to the pan
4. Stir and lift the eggs to cook thoroughly
5. Add ¼ tsp. of bean mixture and 2 tbsp. feta down the center of the omelet
6. Fold one-third over and then the other third; serve hot
7. Repeat with the rest of the ingredients to make more
8. Garnish with feta and salsa

Prosciutto and Fig Salad

Ingredients:

- ☐ 12 cups baby arugula
- ☐ 8 whole figs
- ☐ 6 slices prosciutto in thin strips
- ☐ ¼ cup toasted pine nuts
- ☐ ½ cup fresh goat cheese, crumbled
- ☐ Salt and pepper to taste
- ☐ Balsamic vinaigrette

Method

1. Mix the figs, arugula, nuts and cheese in a bowl with a little salt and black pepper
2. Add enough of the vinaigrette to coat the arugula and toss before serving

Chicken with Sesame Noodles

Ingredients

- ☐ 6 oz. fettuccine, whole wheat
- ☐ 2 tsp. + extra toasted sesame oil
- ☐ 2 tbsp. warm water
- ☐ 1 ½ tbsp. organic peanut butter, chunky
- ☐ 1 ½ tbsp. soy sauce, low sodium
- ☐ 2 tsp. chili sauce
- ☐ 2 cups cooked chicken, shredded
- ☐ Juice of 1 lime
- ☐ 1 sliced bell pepper, red or yellow
- ☐ 2 cups sugar snap peas

Optional ingredients – 1 cup shelled cooked edamame

Method

1. Boil a large pan of salted water and add the fettuccine – cook as per instructions on pack
2. Drain and toss with a little sesame oil
3. Mix the water, lime juice, soy sauce, peanut butter, chili sauce and sesame oil together and microwave for about 45 seconds; stir well to combine
4. Toss the noodles in the sauce
5. Stir the chicken, pepper, edamame and pepper together and combine in the noodle before serving

Crab and Avocado Salad

Ingredients

- [ ] 8 oz. crab meat
- [ ] ½ cup cucumber peeled, seeded and chopped
- [ ] ½ cup red onion, minced
- [ ] ¼ cup fresh cilantro, chopped
- [ ] 1 red jalapeno pepper, minced
- [ ] 1 tbsp. fish or soy sauce
- [ ] 1 tbsp. sugar
- [ ] Juice of 1 lime
- [ ] Salt
- [ ] 4 Haas avocado, pitted and halved
- [ ] 1 lime, cut in quarters

Method

1. Mix the onion, cucumber, crab, fish sauce, jalapeno, cilantro, juice and sugar together stirring to combine – try not to break the crab up too much
2. Salt the avocado lightly and spoon the crab into the halves
3. Serve with lime

Chinese Chicken Salad

Ingredients

- ½ head red cabbage
- 1 head Napa cabbage
- ½ tbsp. sugar
- 2 cups chicken, cooked and shredded
- ½ cup Asian vinaigrette (bottled)
- 1 cup cilantro, fresh
- 1 cup mandarin orange
- ¼ cup toasted almonds, sliced
- Salt and pepper to taste

Method

1. Cut the cabbages lengthways and take the cores out
2. Slice thinly and toss in the sugar
3. Toss cold chicken in the vinaigrette and warm in the microwave
4. Add to the other ingredients, toss together and serve

Peaches and Grilled Pork

Ingredients

- 4 bone-in pork chops, 1" thick
- Olive oil
- Salt and pepper
- 2 peaches, pitted and halved
- 2 tbsp. toasted pine nuts
- 1 small thinly sliced red onion
- ½ cup blue cheese, crumbled
- 1 tbsp. balsamic vinegar

Method

1. Heat your grill
2. Brush olive oil over the chops and season
3. Grill for about 4 or 5 minutes on each side – it should be charred but not burnt on the outside
4. Brush oil over the peaches and grill them, cut side facing down, for about 5 minutes
5. Remove them and slice them
6. Toss the peaches with the rest of the ingredients
7. Spoon the mixture onto each chop and serve

Honey and Mustard Salmon

Ingredients

- ☐ 4 salmon fillets
- ☐ 1 tbsp. butter
- ☐ 1 tbsp. Dijon mustard
- ☐ 1 tbsp. brown sugar
- ☐ 1 tbsp. soy sauce
- ☐ 1 tbsp. organic honey
- ☐ ½ tbsp. olive oil
- ☐ Salt and pepper

Method

1. Preheat your oven to 400° F
2. Mix the sugar and butter together and microwave for about 30 seconds until melted
3. Add the soy sauce, honey and mustard, stirring well
4. Heat the oil and season the salmon
5. Place skin-side up in the pan and cook for 3 or 4 minutes until browned. Flip and cook the other side
6. Brush the glaze over the salmon and place in the oven; cook for about 5 minutes, until the fish is flaky but firm – don't let white fat appear on the surface
7. Remove from the oven, brush more glaze on and serve

Bagged Halibut

Ingredients

- [ ] 2 fillets of halibut
- [ ] 8 oz. marinated and drained artichoke hearts
- [ ] 1 cup cherry tomato
- [ ] 2 tbsp. chopped olives, Kalamata variety
- [ ] ½ fennel bulb, thinly sliced
- [ ] 1 lemon cut in half - half quartered, the other sliced thinly
- [ ] ¼ dry white wine
- [ ] Salt and pepper

Method

1. Preheat your oven to 400° F
2. Place each fish fillet on a sheet of parchment paper and top with an even layer of artichoke, olive, fennel, tomato and slices of lemon
3. Drizzle olive oil and wine over the top, season and wrap in the paper, sealing it up tight so the steam can't escape
4. Bake the fish for about 20 to 25 minutes and serve garnished with lemon

Shrimp and Mango Summer Rolls

Ingredients

- ☐ 1 tbsp. organic chunky peanut butter
- ☐ 1 tbsp. sugar
- ☐ 1 tbsp. fish or soy sauce
- ☐ 1 tbsp. + extra rice wine vinegar
- ☐ 2 oz. vermicelli
- ☐ 8 sheets rice paper
- ☐ ½ lb. medium shrimp, cooked and halved
- ☐ ½ thin sliced red bell pepper
- ☐ 1 peeled and pitted mango sliced into slim strips
- ☐ 4 green scallions, cut into slim strips
- ☐ ½ cup of fresh cilantro or fresh mint

Method

1. Mix the sugar, peanut butter, fish sauce, and vinegar together with 1 tbsp. warm water. Stir well and set aside
2. Cook the noodle, drain and toss with a little vinegar
3. Dip a rice paper into warm water for a couple of seconds, until warm and bendy. Lay it on a cutting board
4. Divide the ingredients into 8 and spread each portion over the rice paper, leaving ½ inch at each end
5. Fold the rice paper ends in towards the middle and then roll it up like a burrito
6. Repeat with the rest and serve with the sauce

Beijing Wings

Ingredients

- ½ cup soy sauce, low sodium
- ¼ cup brown sugar
- 4 minced garlic cloves
- 1 tbsp. fresh grated ginger
- 2 lb. chicken wings
- 1 tbsp. Sriracha
- 2 tbsp. butter
- Juice from ½ a lime

Optional – chopped scallions and sesame seeds

Method

1. Mix the soy sauce with 2 tbsp. brown sugar, the ginger and the garlic in a Ziploc bag
2. Add the wings and shake to coat thoroughly
3. Refrigerate for between 1 and 8 hours
4. Preheat your oven to 450° F
5. Line a baking sheet with foil and lightly oil it
6. Take the wings from the bag and lay them onto the foil
7. Roast for 15 minutes or until cooked through
8. Heat up the lime juice, Sriracha and butter, add the rest of the sugar and stir well to combine
9. Add the wings to the melted mixture and sauté for between 2 and 3 minutes or until the sauce is clinging to the meat
10. Serve garnished with the seeds and scallions if using

Chicken Pot Stickers

Ingredients

- [ ] 2 dozen pot stickers, frozen – vegetable, pork or chicken
- [ ] 1 tbsp. peanut or sesame oil
- [ ] 4 oz. sliced mushrooms
- [ ] 2 cups of trimmed snow or sugar snap peas
- [ ] 1 tbsp. rice wine vinegar
- [ ] 1 tbsp. soy sauce
- [ ] Sriracha to taste

Optional – sesame seeds

Method

1. Boil a large pan of water and add the pot stickers. Cook until soft but not gummy, a few minutes
2. Drain and leave to one side
3. Heat the oil and add the mushrooms, cooking until lightly browned
4. Add the pot stickers and cook until brown and crispy on the bottom
5. Add the snap peas and toss in the last minute of cooking
6. Take off the heat, add the Sriracha, soy sauce, and vinegar, stirring gently
7. Serve with the sesame seeds

Thai Chicken Curry

Ingredients

- [ ] 1 tbsp. canola or peanut oil
- [ ] 1 large sliced onion
- [ ] 2 cloves minced garlic
- [ ] 2 tbsp. fresh minced ginger
- [ ] 1 tbsp. red curry paste
- [ ] 14 oz. coconut milk
- [ ] 1 cup chicken stock
- [ ] 1 sweet potato, peeled and cubed
- [ ] 8 oz. green beans
- [ ] 1 lb. chicken breast, boneless and skinless cut into ¼ inch strips
- [ ] Juice of 1 lime
- [ ] 1 tbsp. fish sauce
- [ ] Chopped fresh basil or cilantro for garnish
- [ ] Brown rice, steamed

Method

1. Heat the oil and sauté the garlic, ginger, and onions for about 5 minutes
2. Add the curry paste and cook for a few more minutes
3. Add the broth and milk, stir and bring up to a simmer
4. Add the potato, simmer for about 10 minutes, then stir the beans and chicken in
5. Cook for 5 minutes until the chicken is cooked and the vegetable are tender
6. Add the fish sauce and lime juice, stir in and serve over the rice. Garnish with the herbs

Sea Bass Packet

Ingredients

- [ ] 4 sea bass
- [ ] 8 asparagus spears trimmed and chopped
- [ ] 4 oz. mushrooms, shitake with stems removed
- [ ] 1 tbsp. grated fresh ginger
- [ ] 2 tbsp. soy sauce, low sodium
- [ ] 1 tbsp. Mirin Sake or a sweet white wine
- [ ] Salt and pepper

Method

1. Preheat your oven to 400° F
2. Lay out 4 large sheets of aluminum foil
3. Fold them into thirds and lay a fillet in the center
4. Scatter mushrooms, ginger and asparagus over the top and drizzle the wine and soy sauce over the top
5. Season, fold the foil over the fish, roll the ends to towards the middle and seal tightly
6. Place the packages on a baking tray and cook for about 15 or 20 minutes
7. Serve in the packets

Swordfish Grilled with Pesto

Ingredients

- [ ] 2 tbsp. pesto, bottled
- [ ] 4 swordfish steaks
- [ ] 1 tbsp. olive oil
- [ ] 2 cloves peeled and crushed garlic
- [ ] 2 cups cherry tomatoes
- [ ] Salt and pepper

Method

1. Smear pesto over the steaks, over them and leave to marinate for 30 minutes in the refrigerator
2. Heat up the oil and cook the garlic of a couple of minutes, or until light brown
3. Add the tomatoes, sauté until the skins have started to blister and season
4. Preheat the grill, season the fish and cook for 4 or 5 minutes under a hot grill. Flip the steaks and cook the other side
5. Reheat the tomato mix and serve over the top of the steak

Grilled Salmon and Ginger-Soy Butter

Ingredients

- ☐ 2 tbsp. softened unsalted butter
- ☐ ½ tbsp. chives, minced
- ☐ ½ tbsp. fresh grated ginger
- ☐ Juice from 1 lemon
- ☐ ½ tbsp. soy sauce, low-sodium
- ☐ 4 salmon fillets
- ☐ Salt and pepper
- ☐ 1 tbsp. olive oil

Method

1. Combine the lemon juice, butter, ginger, chives, and soy sauce together; set to one side
2. Preheat the grill and season the salmon, rubbing oil in as well
3. Oil the grill grates and cook the salmon, skin side down, until the skin is crisp, about 4 or 5 minutes
4. Turn and cook the other side to your taste
5. Serve with a dollop of the butter mix, allowing it to melt over the fish

Spicy Thai Chicken and Basil

Ingredients

- ☐ 1 tbsp. canola or peanut oil
- ☐ 1 thin sliced red onion
- ☐ 2 thin sliced jalapeno peppers
- ☐ 4 minced cloves of garlic
- ☐ 1 lb. chicken breast, skinless and boneless, chopped into small bits
- ☐ 1 tbsp. sugar
- ☐ 1 tbsp. soy sauce, low sodium
- ☐ 2 cups fresh basil
- ☐ Brown rice

Method

1. Heat the oil and add the jalapenos, onion and the garlic. Stir-fry for a couple of minutes, keeping it all moving
2. Add the chicken and cook until it starts to brown
3. Add the sugar, soy sauce, basil and fish sauce, stir and cook for another minute
4. Serve with brown rice

Chicken with Capers, Tomato and Olives

Ingredients

- ☐ 4 chicken breast skinless and boneless, pounded to ¼ inch thickness
- ☐ Salt and pepper
- ☐ 2 cups chopped tomato
- ☐ ½ red onion, diced
- ☐ ½ cup pitted and chopped olives
- ☐ ¼ cup pine nuts
- ☐ 2 tbsp. capers
- ☐ 2 tbsp. olive oil

Optional – fresh basil, sliced thin

Method

1. Preheat your oven to 450° F
2. Season the chicken
3. Lay out four sheets aluminum foil
4. Fold each one in half and then fold up about an inch on each side to make 4 trays
5. Place a chicken breast into each tray
6. Mix the rest of the ingredients together and season
7. Spoon the mixture over the chicken
8. Bake for about 15 minutes and serve with any juices drizzled over the top and garnished with basil

Teriyaki Pork with Apple Chutney

Ingredients

- 4 pork chops
- 1 cup teriyaki marinade
- ½ tbsp. canola or peanut oil
- ½ diced onion
- 1 tbsp. fresh ginger, grated
- 1 cored and peeled apple, diced
- ¼ cup apple cider vinegar
- ½ cup apple juice
- 1 tsp. five-spice Chinese powder

Method

1. Put the marinade into a Ziploc bag
2. Add the pork chops and shake to coat
3. Marinate for between 1 and 8 hours in the refrigerator
4. Preheat the grill
5. Heat the oil over medium heat and cook the ginger and onion for a couple of minutes
6. Add the vinegar juice, apple, and Chinese powder, stir and simmer on a lower heat for 10 minutes – the apples will be soft but not mushy and the liquid should thicken a little
7. Remove the chops from the marinade, soak off the excess sauce and grill for about 5 minutes one each side until charred lightly
8. Serve with the apple chutney

Roast Pork Loin and Lemon Beans

Ingredients

- 3 cloves minced garlic
- Zest from 2 oranges
- 1 tbsp. fennel seed
- 1 ½ tbsp. fresh chopped rosemary
- 1 tbsp. olive oil
- 1 pork loin with a little fat on it
- Salt and pepper
- 2 16 oz. cans of white beans, drained and rinsed
- Juice from 1 lemon

Method

1. Preheat your oven to 450° F
2. Mix the fennel seed, zest, garlic and 1 tbsp. rosemary together on a chopping board. Using a knife, run it through until the mixture feels like a paste
3. Spoon it into a bowl, add the olive oil and combine
4. Season the pork and then rub the paste all over it
5. Either cook straight away or marinate for a few hours for a better flavor
6. To cook, oat for 25 or 30 minutes in a pan until you get a reading from an instant thermometer of 150° to 155° F when inserted into the middle
7. Take it out of the oven and leave to rest for 10 minutes before you slice it
8. Mix the beans with the rest of the rosemary and lemon juice and cook, warming through. Season and serve with the pork and beans

Rosemary and Garlic Roast Beef

Ingredients

- ☐ 3 lb. rump roast
- ☐ 8 peeled and halved garlic cloves
- ☐ 2 tbsp. olive oil
- ☐ ½ tbsp. fresh chopped rosemary
- ☐ Salt and pepper

Method

1. Half an hour before cooking, allow the beef to sit at room temperature
2. Reheat your oven to 250° F
3. Using a small sharp knife, make cuts into the roast, and insert garlic cloves all over it
4. Rub the olive oil over the roast and season with rosemary, salt, and pepper
5. Put onto a rack on a baking tray and cook in the center of the oven for 90 minutes
6. Turn the heat to 475° and roast for a further 15 minutes, or until the beef has turned a deep brown. A thermometer should read 140° F when inserted the middle

Provençal Chicken

Ingredients

- ☐ 1 tbsp. olive oil
- ☐ 8 chicken thighs, skinless and boneless
- ☐ Salt and pepper
- ☐ 1 yellow onion, minced
- ☐ 3 minced garlic cloves
- ☐ 3 diced Roma tomatoes
- ☐ 1 cup white wine, dry
- ☐ 1 cup chicken broth
- ☐ 1 tsp. Herbs de Provence
- ☐ ¼ cup rough chopped, pitted olives, Kalamata variety
- ☐ Fresh basil for garnishing

Method

1. Heat up the oil in a sauté pan
2. Season the chicken and cook for about 6 minutes, turning once. Put to one side
3. Add the garlic, onion and tomatoes, cooking for 5 minutes or so, until the vegetables are soft
4. Add the herbs, broth and wine, bring up to a simmer and then add the chicken back in
5. Simmer for about 20 minutes, uncovered and turning the chicken once
6. Stir the olives in, garnish and serve

Herb Roasted Turkey Breast

Ingredients

- [ ] 8 cups of water
- [ ] 1 cup sugar
- [ ] ¾ cup salt
- [ ] 1 large turkey breast, skinless and boneless
- [ ] 2 clove peeled garlic
- [ ] Salt and pepper
- [ ] 1 tbsp. olive oil
- [ ] ½ tbsp. fresh rosemary, minced

Method

1. Put the sugar, salt, and water into a large pot and bring to the boil, stirring till the salt and sugar have dissolved
2. Allow to cool down to room temperatures and then add the turkey
3. Cover and leave in the refrigerator for 4 hours or more
4. Preheat your oven to 425° F
5. Take the turkey out of the liquid and pat it dry
6. Roll it up so it looks like a log and use butcher string to tie it into this shape, using three knots, each about 2 inches apart
7. Mince the garlic and mix with the oil and rosemary
8. Rub it on the turkey along with some pepper
9. Put the meat into a large pan and roast for about one hour. A thermometer inserted should read 160° F
10. Serve with traditional roast sides

Conclusion

First, I would like to thank you for reading my book. I hope that you found it helpful and informative and I hope that it will be enough for you to realize that this isn't any old detox program. Most detoxes require you to limit yourself to just fruit or just liquid for a few days and we all know that this is not a healthy way of living.

The human body requires a certain level of vitamins, antioxidants, and minerals in order to perform at its best. If it isn't getting them, then there is a high chance that your body systems are not doing what they hold be doing. A "normal" detox may cleanse your body but, because you have been mistreating your body throughout the detox, any weight that you lost will only be water weight and you will pile those pounds (and a few more besides) straight back on when you finish the cleanse.

With the tea cleanse, because you are cutting the bad rubbish out of your diet and you are continuing to eat real food all the way through, your body is given the chance to work properly. The toxins are removed in a much gentler way and your body learns to cope with a decent diet again. It is now able to perform all of its tasks at an optimum level and this means that you benefit from more energy, less weight, less risk of chronic diseases and you will just feel so much brighter.

While the body does have its own detox process, as you have seen through this boo there are many external factors that affect how it works. A build-up of toxins in our bodies leaves our organs unable to cope with the onslaught and that manifests itself in illness and a general feeling of lethargy. Left unchecked, this will continue to build, leading to a worsening of symptoms.

This is why the tea cleanse is the only detox diet you need. The tea cleanse will leave you feeling refreshed and invigorated, clean, healthy and full of the joys of spring. The only thing I will add to this is that, although this is a 7-day plan, you will learn throughout the week how to eat for health. By the end of it, your body will appreciate the fact that it hasn't been stuffed full of toxic junk through what you are eating and it will be better able to cope with the other sources of toxicity.

When the cleanse is over please do not go back to your old habits. Stick with your new healthy eating regime and you won't regret it – you will never look back.

Please consider leaving a review for me at Amazon.com not just for me but to help other readers as well. Thank you and good luck with your tea cleanse journey.

Thank you!

Thank you again for downloading this book!
I hope this book was able to help you get started with this amazing Plan!
Finally, if you enjoyed this guide, then I´d like to ask you for a favor, would you be kind enough to leave a review for this book on Amazon?
Leaving a review allows me to improve it and good reviews mean the world to me.

Printed in Great Britain
by Amazon